# My Poetry Trip Through Cancer

# My Poetry Trip Through Cancer

*A Cancer Journey with God*

## DIANE PARKHURST
*Jan Chapman, Editor*

RESOURCE *Publications* · Eugene, Oregon

MY POETRY TRIP THROUGH CANCER
A Cancer Journey with God

Resource Publications
An Imprint of Wipf and Stock Publishers
199 W. 8th Ave., Suite 3
Eugene, OR 97401

www.wipfandstock.com

PAPERBACK ISBN: 978-1-6667-5158-1
HARDCOVER ISBN: 978-1-6667-5159-8
EBOOK ISBN: 978-1-6667-5160-4

09/20/22

Dedicated to
David Parkhurst, my husband, caretaker and financier of all
my endeavors
David, Daniel, Kayla and Hudson, my caretakers and
entertainment
Jan Chapman, my sister, counselor and editor
Tammy Graham, my niece, private nurse and entertainment

"I can do everything through him who gives me strength."

PHILIPPIANS 4:13

# CONTENTS

# CONTENTS

# ACKNOWLEDGMENTS

David Parkhurst
David Parkhurst II
Daniel Parkhurst
Kayla Parkhurst
Hudson Parkhurst
Jan Chapman
Marvin Chapman
Tammy Graham
Sean Graham

# ABOUT THE AUTHOR

My name is Diane Parkhurst. I am a 56-year-old wife and mother. I have been married to my husband, David, for 32 years. We have two boys, David and Daniel, a daughter-in-law, Kayla, and a grandson, Hudson. I have lived in Midland, Texas for 32 years. I was diagnosed with pancreatic cancer in October 2020. I believe God gave me poetry to help me process all the emotions I was going through at the time. I have written poetry since my teenage years. Living through this cancer journey has given me insight to what one goes through emotionally during cancer diagnosis and recovery. I pray this book helps you during the trials in your life.

# INTRODUCTION

My name is Diane Parkhurst. I am a 56-year-old mother and wife. I have been married to my husband, David, for 32 years. We have two sons, David and Daniel, a daughter-in-law, Kayla, and a grandson, Hudson. In 2020, I was diagnosed with Pancreatic Neuroendocrine Cancer. To say I was shocked is an understatement. During this journey, I ran a gamut of emotions from fear to depression. After a few days of bouncing all around, God started giving me poetry. I believe He was helping me deal with this devastating news through this poetry. I have always written poetry, but this was different. It was more cathartic than my other poetry had been. This is hard to explain, but some day it just poured out of my pen. It was almost as if God was dictating to me. A few times I would have something happen to me and I felt a strong urge to get to my pen and paper. I then began carrying pen and paper with me wherever I went, because God always made something exciting and good happen to me at the most unexpected moments. Even in my darkest moments, He was there! I hope this book conveys His amazing attributes to you. Most of all, I pray that it reveals to you what God wants to give you from My Poetry Trip Through Cancer!

# I.

## MY POETRY TRIP

About midway through my journey, God gave me this poem. I thought it was the perfect title for the collection of poetry God inspired.

"The Lord is with me; He is my helper. I look in triumph on my enemies." Psalm 118:7

I'm taking a trip
Using my poetry
Through this dance with cancer
To help keep my sanity

I'm taking a trip
Not by my own decision
I'm taking it anyway
And seeing it to fruition

I'm taking this trip
I do not want to go
Down this dark path
With my feelings in tow

I'm taking a trip
I haven't a choice
I know God's with me
To give me a voice

# II.

## GOD'S COFFEE ANGEL

I wrote this after an experience God gave me at a local coffee shop
to show me His great love.

"Give thanks to the God of gods. His love endures forever."
Psalm 136:2

God sent me an angel
Straight from heaven above
He sent a young man
To show me His love

In line at a coffee shop
This young man wanted to pay
For my cup of coffee
To help me through the day

I insisted No because
I thought I should buy his
After all I was older
And he looked like a kid

But his insistence won over
All the arguments I made
So I thanked this young man
And cringed while he paid

After we got our coffee
I caught him outside
And told him about my cancer
Letting go of my pride

He said his name was Isaac
And I thanked him again
He worked at a small church
And invited me to attend

He asked if he could pray for me
And I said yes, please
So, in the middle of the parking lot
He asked Jesus to heal me

As I walked back to my car
My eyes filled with tears
This young man I didn't know
Was sent from God to calm my fears

# III.

## BATTLE

I wrote this after a few nights of sleeplessness and waking up thinking of all the worst scenarios that could happen. God gave me this to remind me that I AM NOT ALONE!

"In all your ways acknowledge Him, and He will make your paths straight." Proverbs 3:6

This battle is heavy
On me day and night
It rips me from my sleep
Coaxing me to fight

Is it not enough that
I feel it while I'm awake
Must it steal my night
And cause my slumber to quake

It knows when I'm alone
And at my most vulnerable
It takes my resting time
And turns it insufferable

I pray for day to break
And silence this uncertainty
But then I remember
How to defeat this enemy

To my knees I fall
If continued torment it bequeaths
To God I will turn and call
To protect and defend me

# IV.

## FEAR

I wrote this after yet another night of waking up thinking the worst would happen. God again reassured me that He was in control.

"For God did not give us a spirit of timidity, but a spirit of power, and of love and of self-control." 2 Timothy 1:7

Fear tears me down
With what-ifs and maybes
It throws me into turmoil
Knowing it will delay me

It takes control of my mind
Its intent is to destroy
And render me helpless
So it can take all my joy

Somehow it knows every
Weak crevice in my heart
It knows how to dismantle me
And tear me apart

Destruction of my faith
Is its intention for me
It wants full control
Of my thoughts words and deeds

# Fear

I refer to it as fear
But it has much deeper roots
It consorts with the devil
Its intention is constant abuse

# V.

## FEARLESS

I wrote this after praying to God for Him to sustain me. I believe He gave me this poem to comfort me.

"Have I not commanded you? Be strong and courageous. Do not be afraid; do not be discouraged, for the Lord your God will be with you wherever you go." Joshua 1:9

Today I will be joyful
Without the daily despair
I choose to be without worry
Without doubt without a care

Today I will be a light
Shining for everyone to see
My heart filled with love
Sharing with others God's mercy

I will not be consumed
By a fear that grabs hold
Instead I will only see
That with God I can be bold

Bold in my faith in Him
He will always sustain me
Even when life is hard
Because I know my destiny

It is to serve my Lord
To share my testimony
To tell those without hope
About my Father's story

# VI.

## TROUBLED

I wrote this after a dear friend died of Covid. I was so sad for her children.

"Because you know that the testing of your faith develops perseverance." James 1:3

My heart is troubled
For others I see
Whose trials are difficult
And hard to believe

Their worries are great
And their eyes are full
Of tearful pain
Deep in their soul

Yet they have what
Others desire most
A faith that stands
In the Father Son and Holy Ghost

# VII.

## GLIMPSE OF HEAVEN

I wrote this poem after my quiet time with God and felt the Lord telling me everything was going to be okay! He gave me a peace that passes all understanding.

"And the peace of God, which transcends all understanding, will guard your hearts and your minds in Christ Jesus." Philippians 4:7

You are my refuge
In the midst of the storm
You prepare a place
For me that is safe and warm

It must be a glimpse
Into what heaven is like
A place of tranquility
Without sin or strife

You know what I need
Before I even ask
You have numbered my steps
And laid out my path

So I will praise you Lord
All the day and night
For you calm my fears
And give me your sight

# VIII.

## FRIENDS

I cannot express how much all my friends and family have helped me through this journey. I received cards, texts, calls, food and gifts. The best gift by far is the love shown to me. After starting my blog, I have received so much encouragement from friends. I am thankful!

"Comfort, comfort my people, says your God." Isaiah 40:1

Unsure of my footing
Because of the unknown
Blindly going forward
Feeling I am alone

Seeking my own path
Through this devastation
Wanting peace to come
Ending my frustration

Growing in my despair
Wanting some release
Fearing it may never be
Wanting the worry to cease

Finally I lift my eyes
To my Father up above
Asking for Him to send
An answer filled with love

Then a knock upon my door
A friend I have known forever
Bringing gifts from her heart
This angel I'll remember

Although in human form
I have no doubt at all
That this person here with me
Is an angel sent from God

# IX.

## SKYBRIDGE

I wrote this while waiting for my first appointment at MD Anderson. I had just walked that long skybridge and was overcome with emotion.

"I am in pain and distress; may your salvation, O God, protect me."
Psalm 69:29

It was a long walk
Down the skybridge to MD
The fear in my heart
Starts antagonizing me

I begin to tremble
And tears fill my eyes
How did this happen
And take me by surprise

I glanced all around me
Watching the others pass
Wondering how they feel
And how long my fear will last

I see people with their bodies
Ravaged by this disease
Wanting an answer a cure
And needing a reprieve

I also see people
Who can barely walk
I really want to hug them
And sit with them and talk

My heart breaks for each one
For the pain that must consume them
All the while thinking
This too could be my condition

When I finally sit down
Waiting for my MD
I say a little prayer to God
And ask Him to protect me

# X.

## WITH GOD

My emotions were all over the place during this journey. Some days I was weak and realized my need for God. Some days I was lost and left my God. I am ashamed to say that, but it is the truth. Every emotion I felt was completely raw. Although I was not always faithful, God was always faithful to me.

Jesus looked at them and said, "With man this is impossible, but not with God; all things are possible with God." Mark 10:27

I will be fearless
And fight this fight
I will rely on God
With all my might

I will seek God
Even in troubled waters
And ask for His advice
So I don't falter

I will look to Him
To guide me through it all
Holding my heart in His hand
Never letting me fall

I will be truthful
To others about my journey
Not hiding from them
But sharing it completely

I will not be afraid
To share my emotions
Standing before God
With pure devotion

I will not stand quietly
Before my Father's throne
But boldly go before Him
For I am never alone

# XI.

## GRATEFUL

Today I am breaking from the cancer poetry because God gave me this poem after going to the grocery store and then lunch with my husband. I was so thankful that I was able to do these things that I had to sing God's praises!

Also, I woke thinking about a lady who might help me with health questions. As I was unloading groceries from my car, she literally ran by me and we had a lovely chat. Thank you, God, for planning my day and taking care of every detail! God is awesome!

"Give thanks in all circumstances, for this is God's will for you in Christ Jesus." 1 Thessalonians 5:18

Today I am grateful
Just to wake up
To have breakfast with David
And coffee in my cup

Today I am grateful
For the morning sun
Rejuvenating my soul
When day has begun

Today I am grateful
For taking another breath
And being able to see
God's love in all its depth

# XII.

## DOWNTURN

I wrote this poem after realizing that my way of life would forever change because of the cancer. This particular type of cancer affects how much I eat and what I eat. That seems a small insignificant thing, but I believe satan uses every tidbit he can grasp to bring us down.

"Put on the full armor of God, so that you can take your stand against the devil's schemes." Ephesians 6:11

My heart is heavy
It drags me down
Through thoughts that paralyze
When no one is around

Satan knocks at every door
Waiting for me to fall
And believe his lies
Convincing me of them all

He scurries about in my mind
Busily preparing a place
For me to be destroyed
And watch as I end in disgrace

He grasps me at every corner
Patiently weaving his lies
Tearing me from my God
Turning me into what I despise

A weak and useless one
Who whimpers at any war
Someone who is fragile
And easily ignored

But this battle is not mine
To fight all on my own
It is the Lord who shares
All this that is forlorn

He is my armor
And protects me from sin
He is the strongest of warriors
With my God I will win

# XIII.

## GOD'S FAVOR

This I wrote after a night of anxiety-filled dreams.

The beautiful thing is God ALWAYS has an answer to whatever turmoil satan brings. Anytime I had a bad night, I would just say get behind me satan and God would come to the rescue!

"Then that person can pray to God and find favor with Him, they will see God's face and shout for joy; He will restore them to full well-being." Job 33:26

My dreams they torment me
They take me to the darkest place
Ever torturing my mind
Showing me no grace

All these questions swirl
In my head all night long
Never letting me rest
With no sense of right or wrong

Until morning arrives
God always showing me favor
Singing me a new song
God making me braver

To face my negative thoughts
Unafraid to trod through it
God gives me strength in my heart
And hope that will never quit

# XIV.

## IT'S OKAY

I think God gave me this poem to give me permission to have all the emotions I was experiencing. Sometimes I feel as though I should always be strong, but then I remember God is my strength!

"So do not fear, for I am with you; do not be dismayed, for I am your God. I will strengthen you and help you." Isaiah 41:10

It's okay to have fear
It's okay to doubt
It's okay to feel lonely
It's okay to scream and shout

It's okay to be silent
It's okay to be still
It's okay to embrace sadness
It's okay to feel

It's okay to be angry
It's okay to get mad
It's okay to have sorrow
It's okay to be sad

It's okay to cry
It's okay to let tears fall
It's okay to be weak
It's okay to be vulnerable

# It's Okay

It's okay to be down
It's okay to be depressed
It's okay to let down your guard
It's okay to show others your distress

# XV.

## GOD'S PLAN

I wrote this a few days after I found out what surgery must be done for treatment of this particular cancer. It is called the Whipple and it is extensive. Of course, I googled it. It is never a good idea for anything to be googled. But as I was praying, God gave me this poem. God told me He was in control of this situation and only He knew my days left in this body. God is beautiful!

"For I know the plans I have for you," declares the Lord, "plans to prosper you and not to harm you, plans to give you hope and a future." Jeremiah 29:11

You are moving Lord I know this
Even though I cannot see
The victory is yours already
Your plan is so far ahead of me

Hallelujah for the future
When you bring it to fruition
You say to me daily that
You know of my condition

My doubt never stops you
From saving me completely
You pardon my ignorance
Loving me more deeply

# GOD'S PLAN

Praise you my Great Physician
You have healed me as I pray
I am trusting you Lord
For you take my fears away

# XVI.

## PRAYER WARRIORS

This poem is about the countless people who prayed for me fervently, faithfully and unceasingly. Thank you!

"The prayer of a righteous man is powerful and effective." James 5:16

On my behalf they kneel each day
Before the King of Kings
They lay it down before His feet
Knowing the answer He brings

Their faith is formidable
It's loyal and it's true
Never doubting for a moment
God would always come through

They show their love in many ways
Just wanting me to see God
His light shines brightly through each one
Sent from up above

These angels come in many forms
From young to old I see
Obeying their Father's will
To help bring peace to me

# XVII.

## WHAT IF

This poem I wrote after learning even more about the pending surgery. I was worried how the surgery would affect my lupus. Satan enlisted fear to overwhelm me. But as always, God comforted me. I wrote love letters to those closest to me to make sure they knew how I felt.

"Find rest, O my soul, in God alone; my hope comes from Him."
Psalm 62:5

What if I don't wake up
From this surgery I must have
This thought stays in my mind
What if it all goes bad

What if I don't wake up
And I have no more tomorrows
Will I miss the people I left
And will I feel my sorrow

What if I don't wake up
Will I know what I will miss
Will I be able to watch
And help protect my kids

What if I don't wake up
From this temporary slumber
Will those I leave behind know
How much I love them I wonder

What if I don't wake up
And my body just gives in
Will my friends and family know
In heaven I'll wait for them

# XVIII.

## HAND IN HAND

I wrote this because, after praying, I just did not want to leave God. God reminded me that He goes with me and all I have to do is stay in communion with Him. What a privilege that we have access to the King of Kings all the time!

"Come near to God and He will come near to you." James 4:8

I don't want to leave
Oh Lord I want to stay
In communion with You
I want to be here all day

God I need Your presence
Throughout my entire life
To lean on You in good times
And also when there is strife

I want You when I wake
And when I go to sleep
And all the hours in between
I want you in my keep

For when I am on my knees
I feel invincible
Because I know I am with You
And You are in control

So I am going to take You
With me when I stand
I know You will guide me
As we walk hand in hand

# XIX.

## ANOTHER DAY

Cancer diagnosis can put your life in perspective, at least it did that for me. I was and am thankful for every day I wake up!

"I have chosen the way of truth; I have set my heart on Your laws." Psalm 119:30

The Lord has blessed me
With another day
Will I use it for Him
Or simply throw it away

Will what I do with it
Count and add gain to heaven
Or will I toss it to the wind
And answer the world's beckon

What will I do every day
With this gift given to me
Will I squander this treasure
And treat it carelessly

No I refuse to let
Satan cause me to fall
I will lean on God
And heed His call

# XX.

## MY RACE

I wrote this poem while I was waiting to have a PET scan to find out more about the tumor. I started evaluating my life and what changes I should make for the future. What will I do with the time I have left, whether it be a month or 30 years? Will I use my time to serve God and be a witness to others or squander it? I want to serve God!

"If I were still trying to please men, I would not be a servant of Christ." Galatians 1:10

God guide me today
Lend me Your counsel
Tell me where to go
Don't let me be doubtful

Help me to see others
With Your perfect vision
Not judging anyone
But loving without condition

Lord help me use
The skills You have given
To let others know
What's waiting in heaven

Give me Your peace
And surround me with Your grace
So I can give others
A glimpse of Your face

# XXI.

## FAITHFUL

Faithful came to mind after my morning prayer on this day. I was and am amazed at God's faithfulness to even the smallest details of our lives. During one visit, my sister went with me and we prayed for everything from traffic, close parking and a place for her to stay while she waited. He answered every single prayer.

"But the Lord is faithful, and He will strengthen you and protect you from the evil one." 2 Thessalonians 3:3

Faithful is the word
To describe the one true God
Because He is always there
No matter where I trod

He is with me when I wake
And throughout my day
He is with me when I sleep
And when I kneel to pray

He is with me when I see
The people He sends to share
Their love to help me along
With the burdens I bear

He is with me when
I am not faithful to Him
He even stays beside me
When I choose to sin

He is with me when my thoughts
Are dark and leave me hollow
And when I cannot see
Any joy for tomorrow

My faithful God is with me
Even though I don't deserve it
He stands beside me fighting
And to Him I will submit

# XXII.

## TRUE LOVE

I thought this poem was a good reminder of God's love for us. Even though the weather and circumstances are difficult now, God is still with us and cares for us. I felt and still feel His love for me in all circumstances. His love is the true definition of love.

"Look at the birds of the air, they do not sow or reap or store away in barns, and yet your heavenly Father feeds them. Are you not much more valuable than they?" Matthew 6:26

You are mine Lord
And I am Yours
You hold me close
In You I am secure

You chase away my thoughts
Of doubt and fear
You comfort me
And those thoughts disappear

You move mountains
Before I even ask
You have numbered my steps
With a love unsurpassed

# XXIII.

## KINDNESS

I wrote this after experiencing so much kindness from people at MD Anderson. It seemed every time I turned around at MD Anderson, someone was going out of their way to be kind. I remember leaving the hospital and thinking I wish the whole world could be this way.

"Therefore, as God's chosen people, holy and dearly loved, clothe yourselves with compassion, kindness, humility, gentleness and patience." Colossians 3:12

In this cold world
Of tantrums, turmoil and hate
It's nice to see kind people
Continuing to stay the same

It lifts my spirit
And gives me wings
To see others love others
Instead of just things

It makes my heart happy
And makes me take notice
To see love poured out
To this hopeful poetess

I'm hopeful because
Of what God has given
Each person's act of kindness
Is a little slice of heaven

# XXIV.

## GOD'S GRACE

I wrote this because I was having a little pity party for myself. I had so many questions about what my life would be like after the surgery and if the surgery would be successful. As always, God met me where I was and comforted me. This verse is one of my favorites.

"The Lord bless you and keep you; the Lord make His face shine upon you and be gracious unto you; the Lord turn His face towards you and give you peace." Numbers 6:24–26

These questions I have
Cannot be answered
I seek them out
But I feel abandoned

Has God forgotten me
Or just given up
On this wretched soul
Seeking His love

I am not deserving
Of one little ounce
Of His grace and mercy
It's me He should denounce

I am but a filthy rag
Completely dirty in sin
Unforgiving of myself
Not expecting it from Him

Nothing I can do or say
Could make me any better
Only God's redeeming grace
Can change this sad sinner

# XXV.

## NOT DONE YET

I wrote this poem in the midst of this journey after a friend of mine told me, "You are not done yet." It inspired this poem. I think this applies to all of us in every stage of life. We are never done until we hear the verse below from our Saviour!

"Well done, good and faithful servant!" Matthew 25:21

My life is not over
I am not done yet
God has great plans
That don't include regret

God knows my future
He cares so much
About every detail
Everything I touch

He sees my dreams
And He lets me know
There is a lot more to do
And a long way to go

# XXVI.

## GOD'S FACE

I wrote this while on a plane trip to Houston, after watching people with masks on their faces walk past me. I thought how difficult it has become to show others God's love through masks. Before Covid, I could smile and say hello; now, it seems such a cold world. God reinforced to me that my actions must be my witness!

"As the body without spirit is dead, so faith without deeds is dead."
James 2:26

I know I should show
Others God's face
By the way I act
And how I run this race

But sometimes it's hard
To relay the message
Of God's great love
In this world so savage

There isn't always
An audience willing
To hear what God wants
Much less heed His calling

# XXVII.

## LIGHT

I have always prayed people would see Jesus when they see me. Not that I am consistent on my own, only when I ask God to fill me with His Holy Spirit. I especially wanted to share Him with others during this journey and He gave me this poem.

"In the same way, let your light shine before others, that they may see your good deeds and glorify your Father in heaven." Matthew 5:16

There is a light within me
Though I am not the source
It's from mighty Jehovah
And fills me to the core

This light will stay within me
It will not dim or fade
As long as I ask the Holy Spirit
To live inside me every day

# XXVIII.

## GOD'S HAND

I was in a waiting room at MD Anderson and met a nurse who was recovering from breast cancer. I told her about my surgery. She told me she had a friend who is a nurse in PICU. She then texted her friend to tell her about me and to take good care of me. I wrote this after she left.

"When anxiety was great within me, Your consolation brought me joy." Psalm 94:19

Why does it amaze me so
When God answers my prayers
Why am I surprised to see
When He shows up and cares

Why is it so difficult
For me to understand
That when I am distressed
He sends someone to lend a hand

# XXIX.

## GOD'S LOVE

I had received results on my PET Scan and it showed no spreading of the cancer. I was thankful for that, but my surgery would wait until December 3, 2020. I was upset because I wanted the cancer out of my body now. A friend told me God has picked this date for you. No sooner had she said that than I found out I was the one and only surgery on that day. God is awesome!

"Look at the birds of the air; they do not sow or reap or store away in barns, and yet your heavenly Father feeds them. Are you not much more valuable than they?" Matthew 6:26

I woke this morning
With praise on my mind
For a heavenly Father
So generous and kind

Why should He care
For someone like me
I'm unworthy of His love
And tender mercy

Even when my faith
Is so small and weak
God still knows what I need
Before I even speak

# GOD'S LOVE

His love for me is
Beyond comprehension
Because I deserve
Nothing but condemnation

# XXX.

# AWAKE

I was inspired by the book of Psalm. This was the very first poem I wrote during this cancer journey.

"Awake and rise to my defense! Contend for me, my God and Lord."
Psalm 35:23

Awake my soul awake
From your deep slumber
Of darkness in the valley
And the joy you plunder

Awake my heart awake
From lukewarm madness
From sinking deeper
Into joyless everyday sadness

Awake my mind awake
From evil thoughts and heartache
Just dwelling on the bad
And all the goodness you forsake

Awake my body awake
From the pain you feel
In your bones and pity
You have that makes you reel

Awake Awake Awake
Spend no more energy or time
Fighting this battle alone
For God is with you to fight

# XXXI.

## ANXIETY TRIP

I wrote this before my surgery still fearing the worst. It seems I kept returning to this dark place, but God also kept returning to take me out of it. He is faithful.

"Do not be anxious about anything, but in every situation, by prayer and petition, with thanksgiving, present your requests to God." Philippians 4:6

The closer I get to surgery
The more nervous I get
Anxiousness is here
And it won't let me rest

Thoughts of the worst
Travel through my head
I try to calm myself
But fear returns instead

I'm frightened by the unknown
What will the outcome be
Will I survive it all
Or will this surgery take me

Will I wake from this sleep
Or will I stay in slumber
I can't foresee the future
Will fear ever leave I wonder

# ANXIETY TRIP

I tell myself to be calm
But it has a tight grip
I'll turn my eyes to Jesus
And He will end this anxiety trip

# XXXII.

## STORM

I wrote this poem just trying to get myself ready for this fight. I knew only God could get me through it.

"Hasten, O God, to save me; come quickly, Lord, to help me."
Psalm 70:1

I am waiting for this storm
To fling me into its core
Anxiously waiting to begin
The long struggle and war

Waiting to see what end
Awaits me consumed by fear
Seeking my Holy God
To save me and draw near

# XXXIII.

## THE DARKNESS

This poem I wrote after my diagnosis of pancreatic cancer. I felt fear
and sorrow. God gave me refuge from the fear!

"He is my refuge and my fortress, my God, in whom I trust."
Psalm 91:2

My Lord has a plan for me
This comforts me along
He takes me in His arms
And I know nothing will go wrong

Trying to figure out
If what I heard was real
And how could this happen
And just how should I feel

Quickly my thoughts
Went to a dark place
Wondering how on earth
I would ever recover my faith

Not in God because I know
He will never leave my side
But in my ability to heal
Because I felt as if I died

# XXXIV.

## MY DELIVERER

Even though I experienced sad times, God always brought me back and reminded me that HE is my Deliverer. He has a plan for me, and I will be okay, no matter what happens with my health!

"The Lord is my rock, my fortress and my deliverer." 2 Samuel 22:2

My Deliverer is coming
He is going to rescue me
He is coming with great power
He will set me free

My Deliverer is coming
To lift me up on high
He is my refuge and
With Him I will fly

My Deliverer is coming
He is preparing a place
He won't leave me or quit
Until He sees my face

My Deliverer is coming
He will part any sea
He is seeking me out
He will bring me peace

# XXXV.

## GOD'S ATTRIBUTES

I was literally on my knees when I wrote this poem. Praising God for what He was doing for me every day. God is always good!

"I will praise God's name in song and glorify Him in thanksgiving."
Psalm 69:30

Down to my knees
I fall at Your feet
I praise You Lord
As I begin to weep

I praise You my Physician
You heal me everyday
I praise You for being merciful
In every single way

I praise You God for hope
You grant me daily
I praise You for forgiveness
Every night You give me

I praise You my Shepherd
You search for one lost sheep
I praise You for Your wisdom
In all situations I need

I praise You my Deliverer
Without You I am lost
I praise You my Saviour
For You paid the highest cost

# XXXVI.

## NEVER ALONE

God never left my side during this journey. And if my humanness told me I was alone, God was there in all ways to tell me I was not alone!

"The Lord is with me; He is my helper." Psalm 118:7

Down this path I venture
Not knowing what is ahead
Trusting in my Lord
Instead of the nagging dread

But I am not alone
I have my Lord's refuge
He has provided me with warriors
Their prayers I never refuse

My Lord has a plan for me
This comforts me along
He takes me in His arms
And I know nothing will go wrong

# XXXVII.

## RESTORATION

I wrote this on the plane to Houston the week before my surgery. I was very anxious for many reasons—from getting on a germ-infested plane to passing a Covid test and, of course, the surgery itself. I asked God to calm me and, as always, He did. He is faithful!

"Restore us, O God; make your face shine upon us, that we may be saved." Psalm 80:3

It's getting real
And coming fast
It makes me anxious
I hope it doesn't last

The time is close
To have my surgery
The stress is high
And makes me worry

It's hard to stay calm
In this situation
So many things
To cause frustration

The only solution
For this desperation
Is turning to God
For complete restoration

# XXXVIII.

## GOD'S STRENGTH

When I met with my doctor a day before the surgery, she discussed with me the very worst of possibilities with this surgery. I knew she had to prepare me for everything that could happen, but this really scared me. God was my only way through all of it. He is the Great Physician!

"Be not far from me, O God; come quickly, O my God, to help me."
Psalm 71:12

As I listened to my doctor
My day turned a little sad
I knew about this procedure
The doctor said I have

But hearing all the different
Things that could go wrong
It made me question
If my body was that strong

It made my heart
Just a little sick
To hear what might
Be the worst of all of it

# GOD'S STRENGTH

Once again fear came
To torment my mind
And convince me that
Everything would not be fine

As I think about tomorrow
I am trying to be hopeful
I must lean on God
To make me once again joyful

# XXXIX.

## BATTLE SCAR

I wrote this poem after seeing the wound from the Whipple. The surgery had taken nine hours. The cut was from under my breastbone to two inches past my navel. Now every time I look at that scar, I am so thankful for waking up each day!

"give thanks in all circumstances; for this is God's will for you in Christ Jesus." 1 Thessalonians 5:18

It's my battle scar
And I wear it proudly
From under my breast
To navel it scarred me

This scar is a reminder
On how fragile is life
To not take for granted
And leave all the strife

In a blink of an eye
This life that I know
Can be taken from me
In one single blow

So live your life well
And love all you can
The ones who are dear
And stick to God's plan

# XL.

## AMAZED

I wrote this while in the hospital after I met a lovely nurse named Latanna. She and I shared some of our lives with each other and were connected by our Father in heaven.

And now these three remain: faith, hope and love. But the greatest of these is love. 1 Corinthians 13:13

I prayed with a stranger
In the hospital room today
Her name was Latanna
And her kindness blew me away

She was embarrassed to
Tell me she had a baby as a teen
But I was amazed
At the courage I had seen

As we prayed out loud
For one another in that room
I was immediately in awe
Of watching God in full bloom

I know we each
Got a glimpse of God today
And felt the love of sisters
Singing their Father's praise

# CONCLUSION

This is my first collection of poetry! Sharing my poetry was a difficult decision for me because I am a private person. I felt God wanted me to share it, but I asked Him for confirmation. After my surgery, about halfway through my poetry, a nurse came into my room to talk to me. She was not one of the nurses taking care of me. She had seen me walking around the ward. Immediately after the Whipple, they make you get up and walk around the ward, increasing the times walked around every day. This nurse told me people were drawn to me and I had a light. I must confess at first, I wasn't sure where our conversation was going to go with that comment. I just told her any light from me isn't from me, it is from God. She understood what I was saying because she, too, is a Christian. I shared my story and my poetry with her. She said that I should put this in book form because there is nothing similar available for patients going through this procedure. There it was—the confirmation I had asked of God. Wow! My eyes filled with tears. Even now as I am typing this, I have goosebumps. Man, oh man, God is so awesome!

Once I was released from MD Anderson and safely back at home, I began a blog called mypoetrytrip.com. I shared my poetry on all my social media accounts. The first blog I posted, I nearly had a heart attack because I was so nervous. I was laying it all out there. It was all my deepest emotions while going through my journey. I was sure this is what God wanted me to do. I received so much positive feedback from my friends and people on social media. I received a few emails from my "confirmation nurse" telling me she had shared my blog with others going through the same journey and it had helped them! God is amazing!

Satan did put roadblocks in front of me by way of health issues and that slowed me down a bit. I had been hospitalized several times for kidney stones, surgery complications and bronchitis. My husband teases me saying the ambulance drivers wave at me when they pass by me. Ha. All of the trials inspired my next collection of poetry, entitled My Poetry Trip Through Recovery, hopefully coming soon!

I do not know how long I have on this earth, but I do know I want God with me all the time! I pray this book reaches the people for whom God intends it.